The Booby Prize

My Journey Through Breast Cancer

Bonnie J Wilson

This book is dedicated to my spouse, Michael; my friends Wes and Bonnie Smith who made the journey fun; all my faithful church family that stood by me through the highs and lows; and to God, from whom I get my strength, hope and peace.

Table of contents

Forward

I'm a procrastinator. In fact, it has taken me months to start writing this book. I may be in a nursing home by the time I finish it. I have delved in procrastination since high school. I would wait until the day before an assignment was due and work feverishly to complete it at the last minute. It is just my nature.

Unfortunately, I have let that nature spill over into other areas of my life, including my health. It could have cost me dearly. Maybe I will learn from this journey to stay on top of those things that are important.

When I started my cancer journey, I thought there might be a story to write, but I didn't want it to be a poor me story or a morose story, or even a clinical medical study. I wanted it to be a humorous story. Those who know me best, know I can't do it any other way. I asked people if it was in good taste to do a lighthearted story about cancer and they all agreed that I had the right to do it any way I saw fit. After all it was my journey!

The following pages chronicle my brush with one of the scariest of adversaries, and how I decided not to let that adversary win!

Chapter 1

I am Bonnie, hear me roar!(or, I am strong and invincible)

I'm one of those people that believe that I will be in the best of
health my entire life. I am invincible. I don't care what family
history says, I won't follow in the footsteps of my dad and grandpa
and get heart disease. I won't follow my maternal side and have high
cholesterol. I won't follow my grandma, dad and aunt down the path
of diabetes. And I certainly won't get cancer! I am that one in a
million person that got the perfect genes. Actually, the only gene I
inherited was the Head-In-The-Sand Gene.

I should have had a clue when I was born. I decided to be born
breech with twisted legs and all. I was a sickly kid with lots of
allergies and a nervous stomach. I have fond memories of losing my
lunch when I visited relatives. I'm sure they enjoyed it. I would get
homesick often. While I never broke a bone, I made up for it in little
ways. As I got older, I would get sore throats and break out in hives
for the stupidest of reasons. I had food allergies out the wazoo. Back
then, I got sick, but I didn't get diseases. This point is important
somewhere in this story.

I made sure that I extended this to my dental health as well. When I
was around 8 or 9, I had ten baby teeth removed. In junior high, I
had 4 permanent teeth removed and got the proverbial braces. They
didn't just straighten my teeth, they turned teeth around and pushed

my jaw up and back. Then, when I was nineteen, they told me my wisdom teeth were coming in at an angle and would ruin all the dental work I just had done. So off I went to the clinic to get all four wisdom teeth out.

This was my first experience with how my body responded to anesthesia. It didn't want to let go. It took forever to come out of it! It's years later and I have been to the dentist about once every 25 years. No real cavities to speak of, but you get the gist of my procrastination abilities. I am at the top of my game!

All of this is leading somewhere. Stay with me here. I lived in California from birth to 2005, or 43 years. At age 40, my doctor at the VA Hospital sent me for my first yearly mammogram. I hated the test as I was always very tender in the breast area and being flattened like a pancake was not pleasant. My mammograms were all negative. I also had the yearly pelvic exam. In 2005, my husband, Michael and I moved to Washington State, to the furthest corner of wilderness you could find, far, far from the big city. We had a little clinic, but the nearest hospital and doctors offices were an hour away. My first medical experience in Washington was a Department of Transportation Physical for my job as a school bus driver. I was sent an hour away for that. It was then that I was told I had high blood pressure, which could affect my ability to qualify for this job. I then was sent to my local clinic to get started on a blood pressure medication regimen. Mind you, I believed I would also be one of those lucky people that never had to take medications for their entire life. Scratch that. Here comes medications one and two. I also had a blood chemistry panel done and guess what? High cholesterol and triglycerides. Here come pills three and four. At this point, I was thinking about buying stock in a pharmaceutical company.

I had a pap smear somewhere in the first couple of years which was negative. Fast forward now to 2014. I am sitting at the clinic while my nurse practitioner (I refer to him as my doctor) says in his funny and humble way while shrugging his shoulders, "You know, you really need to get a mammogram, and you really need to get a pelvic exam, and you really need to think about a colonoscopy. After all, you are 52." I knew he was right. It had been 9 years since my last mammogram, and probably 6 years since my last pap smear. And I'd never had a colonoscopy. The mobile screening clinic would be making its last trip to our area in October, so I decided to get on the schedule. It was now July. My screening would be the end of October. All seemed well with the world.

About a week before my appointment, I called the clinic to verify my time and was told 9:30. I guess I thought that was for my blood draw I had scheduled for the same day. I checked in that day and waited for my blood draw. When it was done, I went to the front window and asked when my mammogram screening was and she said 9:30. I looked at my watch and it was nearly 10:00! I panicked and ran out to the mobile unit. Luckily, they were able to get me in after filling out a ton of paperwork. They took me back, and ten minutes later, I was finished. Not so bad! And it didn't hurt since I was now post menopausal and the tenderness was gone. I was told it would take at least three weeks for my results as they had to contact the VA hospital and get my records from nine years ago to compare with the new x-rays. I went home and gave it little thought.

Chapter 2

Bonnie, meet Spot

About a month after my screening, having put the test in the furthest back closet of my mind, I received a call from the clinic. I was told that I needed to have a follow up diagnostic mammogram and ultrasound "because they saw something in my right breast and need to see more, or didn't see something and need to see more." Uh, pretty vague. Being totally naïve to what it all meant I said O.K. (translated "Yeah, whatever") and got my appointment set up an hour away in Colville, during Thanksgiving week. At this point, I was convinced this was fairly routine and there was nothing to worry about. My friends told me the same in a reassuring manor. After all, there was no history of breast cancer in my family!

As Michael and I sat in the waiting room at the hospital, many thoughts swirled in my head. Is this really routine, or did they see something on the screening that suggested cancer? What if it was cancer? Then what? My questions weren't out of fear, but out of my total ignorance. I got called back to a room to change and wait for the mammogram. I was looking around the room thinking wow, what am I doing here? The mammogram was similar to the screening with a few extra views. When I was done, the technician showed me my original screening results on her monitor and pointed out what had been seen in that initial x-ray that caused suspicion. It was all Greek to me. At least I finally got to see what all the fuss was about.

Next was the ultrasound. I am told it is unusual to get both the mammogram and ultrasound on the same day due to scheduling conflicts. I was happy to get it all over with. I wanted answers so I could quit worrying. They had me go back into the original room where I had changed and I sat there for probably 20 minutes while they got everything ready for the ultrasound. The bed I would be on was situated so that the ultrasound screen was straight above me and I could watch the whole procedure. Once on the bed, the technician put the goop on the spot and started pressing and moving the scope around the right breast. I watched the screen, but couldn't figure out what she was looking at. She'd stop and take measurements, and enter numbers into the computer, then resume the test. After a while, I could see the small darker spot she was working on. I don't know how they decipher that spot, but that's what they get paid the big bucks for.

The doctor came in about 15 minutes into the procedure and went over the same spot himself and explained what he was looking at. It was at that time that he started using phrases like "95% curable". I still thought he was talking about IF it was cancer. He showed me the fuzzy border around the spot. I could see how it was different than other spots they had seen in the view. Once the test was done, I got dressed and waited for the doctor to tell me what came next. He returned and advised me that I needed to come back for a core needle biopsy and scheduled me for December 5th. It was then that the apprehension level rose a tick. I was determined to research all these procedures and possible results and get educated on just what they were alluding to.

Chapter 3
Getting to the Point

When finished, I told my husband about having to return for the biopsy. I then went home and told my church family who immediately began praying about this whole ordeal. I did feel a strange peace about any possible outcome. After all, if it was cancer, what else could I do about it but get treatment? Freaking out wouldn't make anything better. My women's ministry leader, Audrey, asked if I would like her to be with me for the biopsy and I said "yes, please". She'd been through one and had much more wisdom on the subject than I. I also pounded the keyboard and investigated mammograms, biopsies, possible results and anything else I could find. I even decided what results would be better than the other and hoped my outcome would be that which I chose, if it was indeed cancer.

The day of the biopsy came. It was set for 2 P.M. so my husband and I headed over to Colville in the morning and went thrifting first, one of my favorite hobbies. I don't know if it was to soothe me or get my mind off the upcoming test, but I was enjoying myself. We stopped off for some fast food and then headed for the hospital. Audrey would be meeting us there. I got checked in and went back to the waiting room. There was no seating available in that area, so we went and sat across the way outside of the day surgery department.

One of my friends that works there wheeled a patient out and saw us sitting in the waiting room. When he returned he asked what we were doing there and I told him about the biopsy, very nonchalant. He wished me luck and went back to work. My name was called moments later.

I was lead right back to the same place I had had the ultrasound. I changed into the stylish hospital gown and sat in a chair until they were ready for the procedure. Next thing I know I was on that same table under the same screen, so I would be observing this procedure also. I was more apprehensive about this biopsy, knowing they would be inserting a hollow needle in place to guide the biopsy device in to the area of the spot and then cutting sections out. Sounded painful to me, but there was some good numbing potion that made it fairly comfortable.

The doctor came in and explained the procedure from the start, and during each step. It was actually pretty fascinating. The only part that was a bit disconcerting was the noise the instrument made when they took a biopsy sample. It sounded like a staple gun. By the time he took the five slices for pathology, it seemed half the spot was gone. It was small to begin with it, but it was about pea sized now. I figured that was positive! He said results should take about 5 days. It was Friday. I thought waiting through the weekend would be bad enough, but 5 days? AHHH.

Before I got dressed, they sent me next door for a follow up mammogram, then returned me to the outside world. My stress level was just a bit higher, but I was calm. I wanted to get home and just decompress. I felt like a nervous pacing father outside a maternity ward for that waiting period. I told Michael to please call me if the doctor called and I wasn't home. I was at church on Wednesday night and checked my cell phone constantly. No message. I returned home, and about 7:30, he said, "Oh by the way, the doctor from the clinic called. He wants you to call him back". I could have floored him about then. I'd waited 6 days, now I was going to have a brain-fry until the morning! I got up early Thursday and called the clinic at 8 A.M.. The doctor wasn't in, but he called me back fairly quickly.

He rattled off some words that took me a bit to comprehend. Invasive Ductile Carcinoma. The only word I heard was carcinoma. I know what that meant. He went on to tell me that they would get in touch with the next facility that I would need in Spokane to get scheduled for a surgical consultation. This was December 11, 2014. I numbly said OK and hung up the phone. It was kind of a shock, but I really didn't react outwardly. I felt a kind of vibration from inside, nearly a light quaking feeling. I didn't cry or fall apart. Just thought about how my life had just changed over three words.

As usual, my next course of action would be to learn everything I could about invasive ductile cancer; causes, treatments. It was then that I learned that the cause wasn't hereditary. It was a fluke of nature, a mutant gene. Anyone could get breast cancer. Wow. What a fool I'd been! I felt blessed knowing that even with my carelessness, it had been caught at a very early stage, although, at the time, I had forgotten to ask what stage! Breaking the news to my family was hard. They knew about as much as I initially did about cancer and I had to explain a lot of details and reassure them that I would be fine. Next was my church family. I needed all the support I could get from here on out; and Michael would be dragged through the whole scenario, like it or not. He turned out to be very supportive through it all, and again I was blessed. The big unknown at this time was finances. How much would insurance cover and how much would I have to pay out of pocket? I'd heard cancer can be very expensive. I started planning to get all the discounts I could and smooze anyone possible to get out of paying full price. That's me. El Cheapo!

After not hearing from anyone for a few days, I called the clinic back and got the number of the facility I would be dealing with next and called them to get my consultation appointment. I would be going to Cancercare NW in Spokane. They had originally given me the south office, but I lived closer to the north end, so I had to track down the right persons. I finally got an appointment the following Thursday with Dr. Wright. I checked Cancercare out on the web and got familiar with Dr. Wright and his credentials. He looked well qualified, so I felt confident he could do the surgery. I couldn't even believe I was going to have surgery having never had anything like this before, other than dental procedures.

My first trip to Cancercare NW was full of paperwork and notebooks, and appointment cards. The place ran like a well-oiled machine. Once I got through filling out the reams of documents, I settled into the waiting room, which had chairs in an L shape along the wall, a table in the center with a jigsaw puzzle under construction, a television and brochure/magazine area off to the right, and coffee off to the left. There was a big reception desk as you walked in that spanned about a third of the room, with aisles going down both sides and off to the left. I looked around the room at the other patients. Most looked pretty normal. A few looked very worn out. I wasn't sure what I expected cancer to look like. I waited about 5 minutes and was called back to get my vitals done and get weighed. Once again, I got to don the usual medical office frock and wait for Dr. Wright. Michael accompanied me into the office and sat in the "visitor" chair, while I sat on the exam table. The nurse came in and did some preliminary computer work, then Dr. Wright entered. He was pretty imposing; tall, shaven head and about mid thirties. I had seen his photo on the website, so was not surprised. He shook our hands and got right down to business. I asked him about my "stage" and he explained I was a 5 out of 9 on some scale, so I equated that with pretty low. He then had me open my gown and as usual, I felt like veal on display. I was thinking about then that modesty had taken a hike once this all started anyway. He stood back, checked everything out and then had me close the gown. He then explained my options, either mastectomy or lumpectomy. Since I was early stage, lumpectomy was the way to go. It is also called breast-conserving surgery. I would also get a sentinel-node biopsy during the surgery to check for spread to the lymph nodes. With the sentinel-node biopsy, they inject a radioactive material directly into the breast about an hour and a half before surgery. It travels from the cancer area to the lymph nodes and highlights the first few nodes going to the armpit. They then remove those few nodes to check for cancer. If none is present, then there is no spread. This procedure would save me from having twenty or thirty nodes removed initially, so I was all for it! We talked over details of procedures, stats, surgery. He told me it was nice to actually talk to someone who knew what was going on! That was all due to my meticulous and thorough research. I wanted to be aware of all my options! Once the office visit was over, I was sent to scheduling to get my date with destiny. Surgery was set for December 30th at the Deaconess Hospital outpatient building in Spokane.

Chapter 4

Cut it out! Or Spot Removal. (I like either one)

My surgery would begin like most, on the day before surgery. We decided to check into a hotel that was just down the street from my destination, and offered patient discount rates. I also had to stop eating x number of hours before I went in, so we had a fine dinner at Outback Steakhouse around 5 pm. I thought that would be enough, as I had to check in at 6:30 A.M. the next day.

Surgery was scheduled for 12:00 P.M. In and out, no problem. Ha! I checked in on time. The lady at the admitting desk offered me a $135.00 discount on my co-pay if I paid that day or within 9 days of my surgery. I considered it and told her we'd get back to her within 9 days. That was a lot of money out of pocket right up front! After check in, I was brought to a suite of rooms if you will, and told to strip, wipe my entire body down with these weird antiseptic pads, put the gown on with the opening in the back, and put those strange sticky socks on. Nothing awkward here. I'm looking at these pads and looking at the instructions, making sure I got everything right. I just knew I would contract some awful disease if I missed a spot. I then sat down on a chair in the room and waited for the next chapter in my exciting, fun-filled day to come.

During my wait, they inserted an IV and input lots of information into a computer and had me sign releases and all that fun stuff. I pretty much sat in the chair until 9 A.M. when they were ready to take me in to put the locator needle in and inject the radioactive material into my breast for the sentinel node biopsy. At this time, I hopped a ride on a bed and got wheeled quite a distance over to the hospital radiation department to first get a mammogram for needle placement. To say the insertion of the needle was uncomfortable was a slight understatement. Once they got it in place, they virtually duct taped it on. There was one final view to verify that the placement was correct. Both the radiologist and technician apologized profusely for any discomfort I may be having. They were extremely nice. My next stop on this whirlwind tour was a very skinny room in which the bed barely fit. It took some precision driving to wedge it in. A few minutes later the radioactive guy with a big needle showed up. He was very tall and imposing (are all these cancer guys imposing or what?) with ice blue eyes. He seemed to be uncomfortable with having to bestow pain upon me, but assured me it would be quick. The procedure included him inserting three needles in the nipple area and raising the skin up each time to get the material into the correct place. The first one didn't hurt at all, but two and three, well…

Once that was done, I was wheeled back to the original room in the "suites". I remained on the bed sitting up. Michael sat and read a book. I tried to read and failed. I was supposed to be going in to surgery in about an hour. The anesthesiologist came in once to tell me they were running behind and would get me in as soon as possible. Twelve noon came and went. Other than a potty break, I had been sitting there feeling like bed sores were rapidly developing. My tailbone was so sore. 1 P.M. came and went. Still waiting. The anesthesiologist came back in to let me know it would be just a few minutes. The anticipation at that time felt the same as cresting the top of a mile long hill on a roller coaster and you were about to see the impending downhill side. Mixed with that was the notion that I hadn't had anything to eat or drink since 5pm the previous evening. Finally, the anesthesiologist came back in and told me he would be giving me medication intravenously. He injected the meds in the tube and they wheeled me out of the room and into the hall. That was the last thing I remembered.

I heard "Mrs Wilson, Mrs Wilson, wake up now". I started coming out of a fog and was so weak and nauseated I could not move. I could hardly open my eyes. I don't remember ever feeling so awful. I had been out for about an hour longer than normal, which I had warned them may happen based on my wisdom teeth ordeal. The difference this time is that I still hadn't had food or drink for almost 24 hours now. I don't do well without food or drink that long, being borderline diabetic. After about a half hour, I was able to sit up enough to get me in a wheelchair and transfer me to the second recovery area. I just sat there and held my head and wanted to cry I was so sick. I was told that the surgery was a success, the margins were clear (they got it all), and the lymph nodes were negative for any spread. I was happy in a sick, half-brain-dead kinda way. The nurse asked if I would like something to eat and drink and, even though I didn't think I could keep anything down, I agreed. I got some yogurt and string cheese and a half can of diet coke, which I sipped very slowly. I could hardly peel the cheese or hold the can up to my mouth. I started to feel just a bit better. They figured I was dehydrated and they were probably right. I was finally strong enough to shuffle to the bathroom and take care of my bladder. I returned and finished off my yogurt and coke. About 20 minutes later, they decided I was well enough to be discharged. The time was 6:30 P.M! I was finally being sprung. I still felt lousy, but at least I could go back to the hotel and sleep. They brought the wheelchair and Michael retrieved the car. I crawled into the car and slumped against the door. The outside temperature was 10 degrees and I had a short sleeve shirt on and my coat was in my arms. I didn't care. Once at the hotel, Michael retrieved a wheelchair from the lobby and got me into the room. I noticed a pitcher of flowers in the room from my friends, the Smiths. How sweet was that? I gave em a good sniff and hit the bed. I had two prescriptions to be filled and the pharmacy was closed. I didn't know what they were for and didn't care. I sent Michael out to procure a pharmacy somewhere in town. He ended up at Walmart. I was in the twilight zone by the time he got back. I looked at the bottles. One was for nausea, the other was for pain. I took the nausea pill and went back to sleep. I wasn't feeling any pain!

I slept as long as I could get away with and still check out of the hotel on time the following day. We needed groceries on the way home. Surprisingly, I was able to slowly walk the aisles of the stores and get through it with minimal hassle. I was still a bit lightheaded and nauseous, but not too bad. The two hour ride home was way too long. I wanted my bed! Once home, we got all the luggage and groceries situated and it was time to pop some pills and go back to bed. The one pain pill was Oxycontin. I had never taken that before. It caused nausea, so I took the nausea pill to offset it. I determined I did not want to take the Oxycontin any longer and used Tylenol from there on out. I felt pretty decent in the next couple of days. I just had to take it easy, not lift anything or basically, not run into a wall with my boob. I would be back in Spokane for a post surgical follow up with an oncologist in the next week or two. We would be discussing my options from that time forward, be it radiation, chemotherapy, or both. It was time to research all my options and be ready to give a thoughtful answer.

During the week after surgery, I had to keep the surgical wound area covered in plastic as to not get it wet during baths or showers. I would cut plastic grocery bags, put one over my head, and tape them shut around my ribs. Showers were awkward, but I made it through with minimum leakage to my dandy cover ups. Some of the bandages slowly started to make their way off, which was fine. I was not going to pull them off! I could not wait to take a shower without that stupid bag on! One interesting side note: After my surgery I craved hot baths constantly. I had no idea why.

About a week later, I went to see Dr. Wright to check on my wounds. He examined them, found them to be healing well, and re-bandaged them. While I am vague on which was my next appointment, I believe it was with my oncologist, Dr. Shri. No one can pronounce her name, so she goes by that moniker. She is east Indian and comes across as confident, intelligent, and trustworthy, not pushy. My bandages were gone and I still had one small part of a stitch sticking out from the wound. I had tried to tug on it, but was afraid I would unravel. I showed it to her. She had a nurse get some scissors and tweezers. She barely pulled with the tweezers and it came out! I felt kind of silly.

Dr. Shri's job was to explain to me my treatment options, statistics, and all that fun stuff. She also referred me to get a bone scan and an Oncotype test, which measures my risk of recurrence based on size and type of tumor, age, and other factors. I have to stop and tell you now, that the Oncotype test alone was almost $6000.00! Thank God for insurance! Dr. Shri asked then if I would like her to draw on the chalk board or if I wanted to take notes. She was going to explain everything to me, past present future. I opted for the chalkboard. She drew what looked like a really long quadratic equation, but it was all very easy to understand. She started with my cancer diagnosis, what it meant, how it can be treated and all the pros and cons of each option. I took a picture of it to remember all that was written.

My next appointment would be with the radiation oncologist on January 15 to discuss what to expect from treatment and procedures to get me set up for it. I was to come back on January 29 to get my bone scan at Holy Family Hospital, see Dr. Shri to get my Oncotype results, and to get measured for my radiation "mold" and tattoos.

It was around this time that I joined an online site called Mylifeline.org. I basically wrote a journal online each day for friends and family to follow my daily goings on during treatment. I will refer to that journal in this book as it has dates, places, times, and feelings that I might not remember by now. The first entry in the journal was dated January 28, 2015.

"Have appt in Spokane for baseline bone scan in the morning Thursday, then appt with medical oncologist and radiation oncologist. I should have a starting date for radiation, and hopefully will be able to set up free lodging in Spokane for the duration of my treatments (6 1/2 weeks). The bone scan is to see how my bones are before radiation to make sure they don't become weakened from treatment."

I showed up at Holy Family Hospital in Spokane for my bone scan. It was very quick and painless and I was on my way to my next appointment at Cancercare NW. I would see Dr. Shri first. She laid out all the statistics regarding treatment and chances of recurrence depending on which treatment(s) I chose to pursue. She gave me my results of the Oncotype test. The low range was 1-18. I was a 19. I felt very confident that I would forego chemotherapy and go straight to radiation as having radiation AND chemotherapy only gave me 2.5% better chance of remaining cancer free than just radiation. I felt the 2.5% better odds did not justify being poisoned by chemicals. I was so relieved! I was also given a prescription for Arimidex, which I would have to take for at least 5 years. It removes the estrogen from my body so my cancer, which attaches itself to estrogen, would not have anything to attach to. It was another way to try and prevent recurrence. I'd read many reviews of the medicine and it could have very nasty side effects such as joint pain, headaches, weight gain, hair thinning, raising of blood pressure, blood sugar, and cholesterol. Those were the very things I was already fighting. I was more intimidated by this medicine than I was the radiation.

My next journal entry summed up the day's appointments.

Finally back from my slew of appointments today. (1) My bones are in great shape. (2) After discussing options and risks, I decided against chemo and will just go with radiation and medication, and (3) Will be set up and "tattooed" for radiation next Tuesday and should start radiation on Feb 9th. Thanks for your continued prayers!

I had met my radiology oncologist that day, Dr. Call. He was a rather short and studious looking guy. So that answered my question of whether all the male cancer doctors were imposing. He reminded me of Benjamin Linus on the Lost Series. He was right to the point and outta there. He was in charge of setting up the tattoo points and exact radiation regiment.

It had been a month since my lumpectomy. They gave me that allotted time to heal before starting radiation therapy. This was when the patient advocate worked with me to set up free lodging 4 days a week and gasoline cards to cover all the trips, as I lived 90 miles from treatment. I also looked into financial assistance for anything insurance didn't cover since I had the 80/20 coverage with the $3000 catastrophic cap. The advocate was very helpful and quick.

At the same time all of this exciting cancer stuff was going on, I was also battling blood sugar issues. I had an A1C test to measure my three month average of blood sugar ratings and it had read 6.0, which is borderline diabetic. Starting in November, I began a low carb diet and exercise routine (anything but sitting still is exercise for me). By January, I had lost 16 lbs and my next A1C was 5.9. I was going in the right direction! I was feeling so much better, not as tired in the afternoons and my feet weren't having nerve pain. I had a lot on my plate and felt like I was juggling chain saws. I knew I would be living in hotels for the better part of 6 ½ weeks and I could not stray from my diet. I would find a way!

The next week, I went to get my permanent tattoo markings, which consist of three dots in a precise pattern to direct the radiation to the exact spot, so as not to kill any good cells as much as possible. The first thing they did on that day was a CT Scan for positioning. The technician was experienced, but he also had a trainee with him. He asked me if I minded having him in there and I said, "oh, no, modesty went out the door a long time ago". He laughed at me. I always crack jokes, especially when I'm a bit uncomfortable. They have a weird "pillow" that they place under you that you will lay your upper body in each time you get radiation treatment. It is contoured to your shape. That pillow is yours for the entire treatment time. For some reason that day, they only put temporary marks on me with green ink and they would do the permanent marks on the 11th of February which was my newest "first day" of radiation. During the week, the marks slowly washed away, even though I was careful not to scrub them or turn directly into the spray. When I returned on the 11th for my first day of radiation, they had to call someone in to do another CT Scan and put the permanent tattoos on. This pushed my first radiation treatment to the 12th. I had already checked in to my first hotel, so they needed to get treatment started.

After my appointments, I went to the store to get a few groceries. I brought an ice chest for my veggies and such. I knew this hotel had a refrigerator and microwave, so I was set for the week. My first hotel was the Red Lion Inn at the Park. It was a pretty upscale place. When I checked in, I was surprised, no, awed, to find out they had placed me in the Executive Wing! I had a king size suite all to myself. All I could think was "way to go American Cancer Society!" I only had one beef with the room. It was a first floor suite and it had an ant problem. I found that out after they attacked a box of crackers, and my dishes, and my sink. I had to drown the whole lot of them and kept most of my food inside the ice chest from there on out. The other disadvantage of this hotel was the parking was $9.00 per night. Oh well, I could handle that! This hotel was in the south end of Spokane, so about 5 city miles or so from my appointments. My radiation would be at 9:00 am and last about 5-15 minutes depending on what was done each day. That left me the rest of the day to figure out how to entertain myself. I'd have to acclimate to living in the big city, a far cry from home in the wilderness. Or maybe just another kind of wilderness!

I met Michael at the hotel and we went to Black Angus for his birthday dinner. We returned and went to the pool and spa for a while. Michael wasn't able to stay overnight, as he didn't bring enough syringes for his insulin, so he went home Thursday night. On Friday I would get my first dose of radiation. I was curious more than anything what it would be like. I had been told that it would cause some light burning like a sunburn and possibly peeling. According to the nurse, I would have to use copious amounts of emu oil, aloe lotion and steroid cream to keep my skin from breaking down and getting infected. I would do whatever it took to come out in the best condition possible.

I decided to enjoy my night, so I threw my four pillows all over the king size bed and sprawled out, turned the TV on and vegged out. I slept great! I felt peace about everything as I knew God was in control of my life, my health, and my future. Whatever he had in mind, I was fine.

The first order of business in the morning was figuring out the best way around traffic to the north end of town. I mapped out a route in my head and gave it a shot. Not bad, about 10 or 15 minutes. I got to Cancercare about 10 minutes early and was sent to a changing room to put on a gown on my top side. There was a separate waiting room just for radiation patients, so I sat there, a little embarrassed, feeling exposed there in my gown. Family members were also there with other patients so I crossed my arms over my chest and sat there and took in my surroundings.

Chapter 5

Feeling that High Pro Glow

The radiation technologist called me back into the treatment room. She and the other technologist were getting my pillow ready and setting up my "numbers" on the computer (inputting the parameters that would tell the machines what to do). I laid down on my back and settled in to the pillow. They put a big rubber band around my feet to prevent me from moving during the treatment. They then had me untie my gown and removed it from the treatment area of my body. They had to move the table up and down and side to side to get me in the precise place. The machine looked like something from outer space. It was large with multiple parts and filled the room. They told me to stay still and left the room. The machine started making whirring and clicking noises with high pitched beeps as it did its thing. They were re-positioning it from another room outside. It would line up to one side and shoot the proper dose of radiation, then go to the other side and shoot another dose in a second site. The whole treatment took between 5 and 10 minutes. The techs came back in, told me I was done and helped me get off the table and retie my gown for the trek down the common hallway. I returned to the changing room and got my street clothes on. That was it for the day! During this time I had entered this into my journal as I waxed poetic that cancer wasn't just about me:

My first weekend home was basically the start of a new routine for me. I started a jigsaw puzzle and also found some to take along with me the following week that could be finished in four days. I had a lot of time to kill in my future. Normally on Wednesdays, I would have worship team practice as I am the worship leader at my church. We worked around it by choosing simpler music and practicing earlier on Sunday mornings. It worked pretty well. I also had my Ebay business to run and was still trying to figure out how to do it on the run. I was using the money I made to help offset the medical costs.

At first, I started putting ads in on the weekends to close the following weekend, so I'd be there to get them ready for shipping on Monday. Eventually, I worked my way up to taking a tote with me that had some clothes to list and shipping supplies. I had my laptop computer and digital camera, so I decided to take the show on the road. I wasn't feeling tired as of yet, so I kept up a brisk pace. Monday would mark my first full week of radiation to come and I wondered how I would feel after 5 treatments in a row. I knew I had hours in each day to fill, so if I needed to sleep, that wouldn't be a problem. I almost felt like my life was a jigsaw puzzle and I was trying to figure out how to make all the pieces fit. I would miss my cat and my home and my friends, and of course, Michael.
Next in the logistics lineup was how to fit everything I needed to take with me in my truck. I had two suitcases, the large tote, ice chest, groceries, puzzles, laptop, camera, purse and jackets. I couldn't put them in the back, as it was winter, after all. It rained a lot. Luckily, not much snow so driving was not as horrible as I thought it was going to be. I tried a few configurations and managed to get everything including myself into the extended cab truck. What fun! I got to bed early Sunday night so I could get up early enough to hit Spokane by 9am.

I would next be staying at the Airport Ramada for the second of 6 weeks. I tried to look at reviews to see what the accommodations were like, but they were all so different, I wasn't sure who to believe. All I knew was that there was a refrigerator and microwave, pool and spa, and they offered a breakfast buffet. I'd have to try it out. I went to my treatment, stopped at the grocery store, hit a thrift store or two and went on to my hotel, since it was a ways out of town. This particular hotel is IN the airport complex across from the rental car lot. It was older, but nice. I was able to request a room next to the pool and spa area so I didn't have to walk across the hotel to get there.

It was a modest room, not luxurious, but very nice. It had everything I needed. When I checked in, they had given me vouchers for free breakfast buffet every morning. I thought I was in hog heaven! Once I unloaded my belongings, which was no easy task, I went next door to check out the pool. It looked inviting. I got changed and went for a dip. It felt good, but hurt my chest area just a little bit when I put my arms out in front of me. At least I was getting exercise. I returned to my room to get some dinner. I had brought salad makings and veggies, so I cut up a big bowl of veggies and had some ranch dressing with them. It was more than enough. I got on the computer, played a few games, worked on my puzzle, watched TV, and went to bed. This would pretty much be my routine for a month and a half!

Chapter 6

A Parallel Universe

This chapter is dedicated to my time spent in Spokane, Washington during treatments. I have never lived in a big city, and my visits are usually quick and amount to a lot of shopping and returning home as quickly as possible. It is a two hour drive from home and a world away! I am using my online journal to help me remember how I spent my time. I already described my first two stays at the Red Lion and the Airport Ramada in a general overview. I tried to take in all the essences of the urban lifestyle while there and make it part of the overall adventure. The following is my life in the Parallel Universe.

Wow, busy day! went to the Goodwill outlet and went "dumpster diving" from 9 to 2. Went back to my hotel room and ate and relaxed. Went and got my radiation done. Went thrifting some more. Came back to the hotel, took a swim and checked out the jacuzzi. My appointments will pretty much be at 9:20 A.M. so the rest of my days are free to explore Spokane.

I should probably explain dumpster diving to those that have never checked out a Goodwill Outlet store. It is a huge warehouse-sized place with large plastic bins on wheels lined up in rows. You start at one end of a bin and ravage through it looking for good stuff. There are household items, clothes, books, etc. I mostly look for clothing as

I managed to get everything home and enjoy my Valentine's Day weekend with my spouse, cat, and church family. My next week would be at the Airport Ramada Inn for four days. I made sure to get lots of rest before returning for a full week of radiation.

My radiation appointments were now at 9:20 A.M., so I had full days to fill. On Monday I went to my treatment then shopped for some groceries and figured I would just go to the hotel. It was the furthest out that I would stay during the following weeks, but still not that far, maybe 5-20 minutes of extra driving each day. My next journal entry summed up the next two days:

Not typing much on here as either the Wi-Fi I have at this hotel is too slow, or the computer is.. I have a lot of delay when typing! Had 4th treatment today and a follow up with doctor and an info session with the nurse on caring for the treated area. Felt a little more tired today than previous times, but O.K. Tomorrow I will be taking a

Ahhh , fun times in the city!! That whole cop chase scenario was so unreal.

The next day, I did indeed visit the Manito Gardens. I remember visiting there when I was young, on a family vacation. I just didn't know these were the gardens until I put two and two together. It was the dead of winter, so I didn't expect to see many flowers, but it was a good excuse for a walk. Even if it was 32 degrees outside. When I got out of my truck, I noticed the sky was very strange-looking. The cloud formations were in a V shape and skittering. Apparently, according to the local news station, it was a rare phenomenon. I felt lucky to have seen it. I walked to each section of the garden looking for any photo opportunities, which were few. Finally I came upon the conservatory which had a beautiful indoor garden display. My camera and I had our way with it and I was done with my adventures for Tuesday. I returned to the hotel and did my usual nap, TV, puzzle, computer routine for the remainder of the day.

I decided that since I was living on the airport grounds, I should go on a people-watching expedition. So Thursday, after my usual morning appointment and lunch. I got my camera bag and set out walking down the road towards the terminals. I thought I was in a ghost town. There were so few people, there was nothing to watch. It was about 1:30 in the afternoon. I walked all the way to the end and found nothing interesting. I stopped at one line and saw a couple of security-type men, one old and one young. I asked the old one if there was anywhere I could go to observe the planes close up and he barked at me that I would have to go to the five story parking structure across the way to see the planes. I graciously said "O.K., thanks" even though I really wanted to tell him he didn't have to bite my head off!! I made my way to the top of the parking structure and had a view over the terminal building of the planes. They still seemed far away, even with a zoom lens. I took a few shots of planes that had been painted with college team logos, a few take offs and landings and a few of people milling around outside. It was really a bust! I walked back to the hotel and took it easy the rest of the day.

The following is Friday's journal entry:

Was really tired after treatment today. It was a looooong drive home. Just wanted to take a nap! I think I had a meeting today to go to, but just couldn't go another mile or minute. After getting everything unloaded from the truck and cleaned out of the living room, I was pooped! Will be staying at the Holiday Inn Express next week. Kinda cool getting to check out all of the accommodations around

After another semi relaxing weekend, it was back to the grind again. It is now the last week of February. I've been very lucky that, while it has been very chilly, it hasn't snowed much making my trips much easier than they could be. I decided to go straight to my hotel after my appointment on Monday and see if they would let me check in early. I had so much junk in my truck, I just wanted to unload. This would be my first week hauling Ebay items with me to try and sell on the go. Thankfully, they did let me in early. I got a third floor room by an elevator and they had a self serve luggage cart. Once I got all settled in, unpacked, computer set up and checked out my surroundings, I had to figure out what I wanted to do for the week. I knew some thrifting would be thrown in, but there had to be some other amusement!

This hotel was my favorite so far. It had all the things I needed in the room, but it also had free full breakfast, free light dinner and cookies, and free parking! I only had to worry about furnishing my own lunch, so I brought much less food. One of my favorite thrift stores was across the street and Riverfront Park was to the north. Michael came down and joined me one day and we walked all over that park, perused a large book store and he posed on the giant Radio Flyer wagon. It was great exercise and just on the cusp of brisk outside. The next day I made a beeline to the breakfast area to check out the pancake making machine only to find it out of order. Boo Hoo! I was so looking forward to it. The other available fare was good, so I made sure to have a decent breakfast before radiation. I was feeling exhausted, so much that my head was swirling. Not sure if it was from the radiation or the insomnia. I would be attempting a nap later in the day. I would also be listing eBay ads from my laptop for the first time. It will be interesting to see how that works out.

From my blogs on February 26 and 27, 2015:

Tomorrow is the last radiation session of the week. It will be #12 of 33. 4+ more weeks to go living like a nomad, albeit not in a tent! Had a great visit today with Bonnie and Wes Smith. They took me to lunch and we had a nice long chat. I took Bonnie to see what all the thrifting hype is about. It was probably overwhelming!   Listed lots of things on ebay today. Have actually sold some things this week that were listed "on the go"! It's not as hard as I thought it would be. Anyway, looking forward to being home again, even if it's only a couple of days. I'll be dropping my truck off for an oil change and walk to my appointment tomorrow. Hoping to then get out of town ASAP! Curious to find out where I'll be staying next week. Have to call the Cancer Society tomorrow.

Finally home and very tired. Pretty much been glued to the recliner since I got home and unloaded everything. Next week I'll be at the Davenport Tower. I will be like the redneck out of their element for sure! Total luxury. I'll be parking a couple of blocks away since they charge $15.00 per night for parking. There is no fridge or microwave, so I'll be taking our ice chest that plugs into the wall for *my refrigerator. No heating up food though, so I'll have to rethink what I'm going to eat. Can't afford their dining options. It will be fun to check out a ritzy place though!*

I found it weird driving into the hood today. I feel like a stranger in my own town!

My next trip to Spokane had an exciting agenda. Besides the ever - adventurous radiation appointment, I would be dropping my entry off at Rosauer's Store for a grocery giveaway, and washing my truck. What a day! I wonder if I'd actually get either of those done! I will, however, get my first up close and personal look at the Davenport Tower. I can't believe I am going to stay there for free (plus the additional cost of parking).

I found my way to my appointment and on to downtown Spokane to the Tower. I had to park at the valet door and figure out how to get my truckload of stuff to my room on the 16th floor. Normally, they would have a bellhop load the cart and take it for you, but I didn't want to spend any extra money on tips, as I am the world's biggest cheapskate. I started unloading my truck and carrying the biggest load I could to the elevator through the door and around the corner. After two trips, the valet guys felt sorry for me and loaded the cart and took the rest up for no charge. I was ever grateful! After all was unloaded, I went a few blocks away to the Parkade structure, which from what the sign said, I thought was $8.00/night. It was worth the walk back and forth in 28 degree weather. Unfortunately, I found out the next day it was $16.00 per night. Not sure how I messed that up, but from then on out, I would be parking in the Davenport structure for $15.00 per night. At least it was right across the street.

Now, as for the accommodations, the room was very luxurious and decorated in safari motif. It had mirrors across the back of the bed with lights, a nice leopard print chaise lounge and a huge walk-in shower. I was overlooking the south side over the railroad tracks and the power plant steam pipes and old brick buildings with the original writing on their sides. It was so totally urban, I could just scc photo potential everywhere! I had a king size pillowtop bed with four pillows. I hoped I could have a great sleep that night! I set up my newest puzzle on the extra table and the laptop on the business desk, unloaded my next batch of clothes to list on eBay and put everything in its place. I knew I was out of my element when I kept hearing a noise like a doorbell. I finally went to the door and there was a maid waiting to turn down my bed. Mind you, it was around 4:00 PM. I said no thanks, but when she offered me some cookies, I said "sure, thanks", and took them and shut the door. I'm not positive, but I probably was supposed to tip her. I just didn't know how to "be" in this atmosphere!

About mid week, I decided to do something I hadn't done in a very long time. I had my long, straight hair cut into a nice, short bob. I also colored it medium ash blonde. When all was said and done, I took a selfie and published it on Facebook for all to see. I hate selfies, but I thought it was time to just do it! Having cancer can make you rethink your fears and doubts and give you courage to do things you normally wouldn't. That was one positive aspect of this whole ordeal. The following week, I would be staying back at my favorite Holiday Inn Express. I posted this blog on March 10, 2015:

Had treatment 19 of 33 today. Burn areas still itch, but they will be giving me a steroid cream to put on them to help keep the skin from breaking down. Next week I get a new CT Scan to make sure the area they are doing is fine tuned to target a very precise area. Like my room this week. Has 2 queen size beds. One to sleep in and one to throw everything else on. Their super quick pancake making machine is working too, so I got to check it out this morning. I lost track of how many sirens I've heard today! Busy city!
Taking it easy the rest of the day. I got a big hunk of my "pizza" puzzle done yesterday, so I am going to dig in today and get another hunk done. Too bad it's not scratch n sniff! Lol

This time I got to choose which floor and what side of the hotel I stayed on, so I took a fourth floor facing south for a different view. I could still see that blasted thrift store, but could also see Riverfront Park and the busy traffic down below. This week, after Bonnie and Wes took me to lunch yet again, I took them to the Goodwill Outlet to introduce them to the fine art of dumpster diving. We spent a couple of hours there while I shopped for more stuff I didn't need, and Bonnie grabbed some vintage books that she loves to read. I think Wes was probably shaking his head and wondering what he got himself into!

I am having trouble sleeping between the radiation burns itching, insomnia, and hot flashes. I kick off the covers, then the air comes on and I pull them back on. Guess I will need to get some sleeping pills before I turn into a zombie.

My next blog sums up the home stretch. It is dated March 14, 2015:

Eleven more treatments to go! I know where I am staying for the rest of them. Double Tree Inn Hilton this M-W and then Super 8 in the Valley for Thursday night. Michael will come down and we can have my free "birthday" steak dinner, then he can stay without having to pay parking. The Double Tree is 12.00/night parking! The last full week will be at the Red Lion Riverfront across from the other places I've been staying, a stone's throw from the Arc thrift store, and best of all, free parking and has a fridge and microwave so I can eat in. I will have the last treatment on Monday the 30th, so we can both go down, do some shopping and go home. Not sure what comes after radiation, but I believe it is just followup from there on out to make sure cancer hasn't come back anywhere. I am getting ready to schedule my colonscopy too, but have to check with my radiology oncologist to make sure I can have that done while undergoing radiation. I will have then been checked for all the major internal cancer types.

This turned out to be an interesting week. After my appointment on Monday morning and a quick trip for groceries, I headed towards the Doubletree Inn. This hotel is located next to the Spokane Convention Center on the opposite side of Riverfront Park from the Holiday Inn. Very classy and normally pretty expensive. I pulled up and parked so I could check in and noticed a police car next to me. I wondered why they were there, but dismissed it as I entered the hotel. I finished my check in and the bellhop loaded my mountain of gear onto his cart and headed towards my room. I believe I was on the 14th floor for this stay. My room had windows facing north, east, and southeast. The views were gorgeous, overlooking the Spokane River and the busyness of the city. I could look down on the bikers and runners along the park path and the landscaping workers. I settled in and got on my laptop computer on Facebook and quickly found out why the police had been at the hotel. Apparently a man had carjacked someone in the midtown area, ditched that car and carjacked one of the Doubletree Inn courtesy vans! He eventually abandoned that and was caught. The same day some guy was out in front of the convention center taking off his clothes and throwing them at cars in line at the traffic signal. I immediately thought, oh geez, I have to park in the parking structure which is NOT attached to the hotel. I would have to be extra vigilant walking back and forth between there and the hotel. I decided to park along the back row so I would be nearest the landscapers and there would always be people milling about. It worked quite well for the week. I managed to escape any potential muggings!

On Friday, I had to move to the Super 8 Motel across town in Spokane Valley. My husband joined me so we could have my belated free birthday lunch at Black Angus nearby. The Super 8 is in a super busy area for traffic and maybe not the best neighborhood. I have stayed at Super 8's many times and found them to be pleasant, average rooms. This motel was by far the dingiest and oldest room I had ever stayed in. The carpets were worn and dirty and the bed definitely was not pillow top. I knew then that this whole experience had spoiled me for the motels I was used to staying in. I'm not sure I could look at an economy motel the same way ever again. I reminded myself that this was free and not to be ungrateful. It was only one night, it had the fridge and microwave and free parking and my spouse could stay with me for free.

I'd be getting a CT scan the next Wednesday and scheduled a colonoscopy for April 9th. Michael would have to take me to that appointment as I would be under the influence of drugs afterwards. This would be my final test for the big three cancers; breast, cervical, and colon. I was hoping to only be 1 for 3!

My next blog was from Wednesday, March 18, 2015. I entitled it "Reality Check":

I was at my radiation appointment early today as I had to have a CT scan first. I was sitting in the waiting room with the other patients that had appointments before and after me. One lady there being treated that is close to my age, Suzanne, was sitting next to me. Another lady I didn't know asked her about her cancer. She said that she had her skin open up on one of her burn areas last night. Then she talked about how she had just finished 7 months of intense chemotherapy for multiple cancers, aimed at shrinking all her tumors including ones in the breast, lungs, bones, etc. She talked about how sick the chemo made her and that she couldn't eat. I felt like I had no reason to whine about my burns and itching after what she had gone thru. I can't imagine if I had to do 7 months of anything that would be 2 hours away from home. My 6 1/2 weeks away are almost done and I will be very happy!

I've seen an impressive amount of positive attitudes in those I've spoken with. It would be easy to have a pity-party over all of the inconvenience that cancer causes. I rely heavily on my faith in God. I pity those who don't have hope in Christ. I can't imagine the fear that must be ever lurking in their lives. It would be easy to be angry and say "why me?" But really, why not me? God has every right to allow this in my life. I hope I don't waste this experience. He obviously has plans for me that I am in training for! The thought runs through my mind many times a day "what if this comes back?" "What if it comes back even worse?" How will I deal with it? I pray that it doesn't. God is there to hold my hand no matter what happens. Time for bed and hopefully, sleep comes tonight. Please keep me in your thoughts and prayers. They will be intensely targeting the area where the tumor was for the last week's worth of treatments. This is also where the fatigue can really hit hard. The drive home on Friday can be a real bear when I'm tired! Also, thanks for all the cards and

I really admired Suzanne. She was holding her head up and not letting cancer beat her! I'm sure she could write a book about her experiences too. There are so many thoughts and emotions that swirl around in your mind when you're going through treatments for a beast you never thought would get a hold of you. I hope she had all the support from friends and family that she needed. I hope she knows the God who cares.

Once again, I made it home for the weekend. I got to see my kitty. I missed her so much! I had cooking class at 2 P.M. so I decided to try a nap. It lasted 15 minutes. Oh well, sleep is overrated anyway. We made chocolate cake from scratch. Yummy! I don't know how I found the strength to be there after only 4 hours of sleep, but I wanted to be there around all my friends and support.

Six more treatments to go. I would be staying at the Red Lion Riverfront Hotel the next week. It is right across the parking lot from that same thrift store! It had the fridge and microwave and free parking, so I'd be glad for that.

My next blog was from that following Monday:

Today was most interesting. Started a new radiation regimen for the last 5 treatments that targets the tumor area. First they took a full body X-ray as I laid on the table. Then they started the treatments and the table would turn this way and that and the machine would

I had Michael ride in with Bonnie and Wes on Thursday so he could
drive me home on Friday. The fatigue hit me hard with the focused
radiation. The pain wasn't too bad. I would have one more treatment
on Monday and that was it! I was looking forward to getting on with
the healing process. I would have a follow up appointment in about
30 days or so to make sure I was healing properly. The following
was my blog on the day of my last treatment:

I can't even begin to explain the relief of that final day and knowing that I could get back to my normal routine. While living in the city was an eye opener, I was ready to go back to my wilderness. This is my last blog related directly to the radiation treatments. It is dated April 3, 2015:

Obviously not a lot going on since my last rad treatment. I find though, that I have trouble focusing on things that need to be done and remembering engagements, sorting through my church activities, medical appointments and all other things and remember what is what and when. Guess I will have to break down and glue a calendar to my forehead. It's a bit unnerving for someone who used to have a photographic memory to admit I just can't keep it all straight in my head anymore. Hope this will get better as I heal and get out from under the effects of radiation. I'm really hoping it isn't the Arimidex I'm taking, cause I'm stuck with that for at least 5 years!

The burns are "healing" nicely, i.e. some peeling going on. Some of the discoloration may be permanent. Don't really care one way or the other. Just don't want to see any more cancer cells taking up residence in my body. Still adjusting to being home full time and getting back into the swing of things. I am sleeping a bit more than I usually do, but that is O.K.. That will change too. Just glad to be done!

Now that I was done with the breast cancer treatments, my focus turned to the upcoming colonoscopy. Getting a passing grade would give me peace of mind so I could focus on the next 5 years of cancer freedom. My appointment was changed to a week later than the original date. My blogs relating to the colonoscopy tell the story from beginning to end, so I'll let them speak.

April 13:

Today I start my liquid diet in preparation for my colonoscopy tomorrow. Drink only clear stuff. Drink some more. Take some laxatives. Try to get through photography class without running up and down the stairs 20 times! Drink tons of Gatorade and Mirelax to clean out my pipes. Drink some more tomorrow and then try to make the two hour drive to Spokane without stopping endless times for potty breaks! Should be fun! I'll be glad to get this over with though, so I have peace of mind that there are no other cancer issues in my body. Won't have to repeat this for 10 years if it is negative. I'll be in the twilight zone from the time the colonoscopy starts until probably halfway through Wednesday. Me and the cat will be napping together....

April 15:

Got thru the colonoscopy. Didn't have any problems making it to Spokane, no extra stops needed. I was soooooo hungry. Hadn't eaten anything solid since Sunday night and by the time the colonoscopy actually begun, it was after 1 pm Tuesday! I made sure Michael had a Subway sub waiting for me when I got done! They conked me out and I don't remember much except they said I might feel something when they 'turned a corner' with the colonoscope. I remember saying "ouch". I woke up near the end of the procedure when they removed two polyps from the rectal area. They were 12mm in size. I will hear from them in about a week on the pathology. Will probably have to get another colonoscopy in three years due to the presence of polyps. The sub was awesome! Spicy italian with siracha sauce, pepper jack cheese, and jalepenos. Probably not the best thing to eat after all that time without solid food, but it was so worth it. Lol

May 1:

Colonoscopy results were negative. That is good. Have to return in 3 years for another one since I had polyps. Was feeling pretty icky yesterday so had Michael check my blood sugar after dinner. It was over 220! Too many carbs lately. I have to get back on to my eating schedule that I had pre-cancer and drop another 10 lbs at least. The Arimidex I am taking can contribute to high blood sugar as well as high cholesterol and high blood pressure, all of which I am already fighting against. Will have to fight harder. Decided to have a high antioxidant smoothie for breakfast to kick things off. Next cancer check is in 3 months. Everything looks good for now.

That was my last entry on my blog. I closed that chapter of my life and entered the realm of post cancer survivalism.

Chapter 7
The Whole Enchilada

I felt I would be doing a disservice if I didn't cover the entire scope of cancer. This would include its effects on the physical, mental, emotional, relational, financial and spiritual aspects of life after cancer and its treatments. I think most people focus on the physical and mental, but not so much on the others. I will dissect how these relate to me and my own experience. This is by no means an exhaustive list. First up would be physical. Remember, this is MY experience, others may have more or less effects.

Physical Effects of Cancer

Where do you start? For me, I had no idea I had cancer until I had a mammogram and subsequent testing. I had no symptoms at all. If you want to include the testing, then the first real physical effect was the core biopsy. Although I was mostly fascinated by it, I was a bit uncomfortable. They numb the area to be biopsied, then stick a filament that reaches from the outside to the cancer spot. They then insert a contraption I can't name and they start taking slices of the tumor one at a time. Each time they take a sample it sounds like a staple gun and feels like a thump. Then there is the stress of waiting for the results.

Once you have been diagnosed with cancer, you meet with a cancer surgeon to set up your surgery appointment, which for me was set up within 20 days of my diagnosis. On the day of surgery, you will have been fasting for at least 14 hours. That is not bad unless your surgery is delayed. You sit in a hospital bed for hours until they finally wheel you back. Thankfully, you are in la la land during the event. For me, waking up from the surgery was by far the worst physical aspect. I was very groggy, very hungry and felt sicker than I'd ever felt. I could hardly move. Once they were able to move me to the secondary waiting room, I was able to take food and drink in little sips and bits until I re-hydrated. I felt well enough to shakily stand up and use the restroom and get in a wheelchair to go home to my hotel. Once there, I just wanted to sleep. The next day, I felt tired, but well enough to get through grocery shopping and the two hour drive home.

I don't recall having that much pain from the surgery locations (tumor and lymph nodes). Maybe some stinging once in awhile and a little discomfort. The real fun began when I started my radiation therapy and began my regimen of Arimidex. Radiation's two biggest side effects are burning and fatigue. I got em both. The treatment itself does not hurt, but it slowly gives you a sunburn over that sensitive area. I'm not sure if the fatigue was just from the treatment, or stress, or anxiety, or a mix of it all. The Arimidex medicine has three major side effects: Hot flashes, joint pain and insomnia. Just what I needed. More fatigue! I did not get bad joint pain, just enough to know it was there. The hot flashes and night sweats have been my enemy! Overall, my anxiety over taking this medicine lowered after I found that I could indeed survive the side effects.

Once you have finished all your treatment and go into "survivor mode", things gradually change in many ways. Having taken so long to write this, I have had a chance to experience the aftermath. I have insomnia from the medicine, which leads to feeling pretty tired and unmotivated. I have sporadic joint pains. I get stinging sensations in my surgical area where the scar tissue is forming. I now have spasms in my right rib area where scar tissue has adhered to my chest. I get pains in my legs, but I'm not sure if that is related to my medicine. For the most part, I am in every day mode. I live with whatever comes. If you remember, at the beginning of the book, I stated "I get sick, I don't get diseases"? My new mantra now is "I don't get sick, I get diseases"! It's true! I rarely get "sick"!

I have lost thirty pounds. My A1C is back to almost normal. I was diagnosed with diabetes, but it is under full control with diet and walking 1 to 2 miles per day. This *will be* my new normal.

Chapter 8
Mental Effects of Cancer

For me, the most irritating effect of cancer mentally is the "what if's". Once cancer has invaded your body, you have no way of knowing if it is coming back. You do all the procedures, take the medicines, eat healthy and exercise, but there is no guarantee. I wanted to nip that one in the bud immediately because it served no purpose. For me the biggest fear of cancer's return is that I already know what I went through once and, well, I don't want to go through it again. I am also of the belief that subsequent treatments will be harsher. I would probably have to go the mastectomy route and chemo, both which I dodged the first time. I'm sure I have it in me to survive it all a second time, but I don't want to!

The second aspect of the mental effects is radiation/chemo brain of what I call "Fog-Brain". Again, having stalled long enough while writing this book, I am now three years out and still have problems with short-term memory. I will start to describe something and the right word will be right there, but I can't get it to come out. It usually takes a minute or two for me to finally finish my thought. I still don't keep engagements straight and have not given in to the calendar. I really need to write things down! I'm very stubborn on that point. Names are fading into the recesses of my mind. Sometimes I can't get motivated to do the simplest things, like work on my Ebay business. There really is a line of demarcation called B.C. Before cancer and after cancer, just like a calendar.

The third aspect of the mental effects of cancer is (as I am writing this sentence, I just forgot what I was going to write). Oh, yeah. It is deciding how you are going to allow cancer to affect your life. Are you going to curl up in a corner and say "poor me?" or are you going to fight with all you have? Being proactive is the best thing you can do for yourself and those around you. It is healthier and more productive. I will cover some of that productiveness in the financial section.

Chapter 9
Emotional Effects of Cancer

The emotions are very closely associated with the mental aspects. But where emotions deviate is in the day to day living through the cancer experience. One day you can be happy and positive and the next day you can be down in the dumps and you feel like giving up.

A lot depends on what aspect of your treatment you are going through. My first emotional response probably didn't appear until I had the biopsy and had to wait almost a week for the results. I was a complete mess until I had my answer. Believe it or not, I didn't care what the answer was, I just wanted an answer! Once I was told I have cancer, I didn't cry. Instead, resolve set in. I would learn all I could about procedures, find out what the next step was, and start figuring out the financial and scheduling impacts on my life in general. That determination stayed with me through all phases of treatment and is still with me.

The first big hurdle was the surgery. I had never had surgery of any kind other than some dental work up to this point, so it was all new and kinda scary. I started prepping at the hospital at about 9 in the morning for a 12 noon surgery and didn't get wheeled back until after 1 P.M. I hadn't eaten since 5 P.M. the night before. I didn't realize that I was getting dehydrated, and also my hind quarters were really sore from sitting on the hospital bed so long. Coming out of the surgery was horrible. I think to this day, it was the most horrible part of my entire experience! I felt lousy, tired, and just wanted to be home in my own bed. The healing process was pretty quiet and the follow up appointments were mostly to decide on my next step of treatment. I was determined NOT to have chemotherapy! That was a decision that I had to live with and I hoped it was the right one. The not knowing if my decisions were right was difficult.

Next, I had to gear up for living in the city for the better part of 7 weeks, away from my husband, cat, friends, church family and my rural home. I had to see it as an adventure, or it would become drudgery. Once your treatments come to and end, there is that sigh of relief, but still some reservation, what with medicines and follow up appointments and healing. Mostly the emotional aspects will be affected greatly by your ability to stay positive and lean on your significant others and friends. Don't go it alone!

One thing that I realized as time went on is that I was going through a grieving process. Grieving for the loss of a part of me, even if it was cancer, it was still my body. Grieving for a loss of my mental faculties as they had previously been. Grieving for my health in general. It helps to realize this so you can go through the steps of anger, denial, and acceptance, just as you do when losing a loved one.

Chapter 10
Relational Effects of Cancer

Relationships can either fail or strengthen during cancer treatment. It goes along with emotional effects, you can make it work or make yourself and everyone around you miserable. I chose to lean on my friends for companionship and strength. Pushing those away that can help you the most can leave you standing alone when you need them most. I had my husband and a friend go to my follow up mammogram, ultrasound and biopsy. Just having someone there to talk to helped. Even better if it is someone who has been through cancer. My family offered to help in any way they could. My friends also rallied around me with encouraging notes and hugs. Of course, Michael was there with me for the surgery and follow up appointments. The only time I went it alone was during the radiation treatments, because I was two hours away from home and had to stay in the city. Michael did come and stay with me in the hotels a couple of times. And of course, Wes and Bonnie took me to lunch and we had adventures together to break up the monotony. Having someone to lean on is so important, I can't stress it enough. The only time I would say to push someone away, is if they are "toxic" or negative and not up-holding to you. A Good attitude goes a long way.

Chapter 11
Financial Effects of Cancer

One of the first things you think of when you get the big "C" diagnosis is "oh, no, this is going to cost a fortune, what if? What if? What if? If you have no insurance, it can be even scarier. I was fortunate to have insurance. If you don't, I would imagine you would have to apply for state aid. I've also heard horror stories of insurance companies refusing to pay for certain things and some have canceled policies because you cost them too much. I briefly thought about that aspect, but I was more apt to start researching all my options to soften the blow and be able to afford what insurance didn't cover. As soon as you set the whole cancer treatment wheel in motion, do your homework! I can't stress this enough! Once I stepped foot into Cancercare, I was hooked up with a patient advocate. They are there to get you help in any way possible. The first thing I had to get covered was my fuel costs for driving the four hour round trip to my appointments. I was given two free $50.00 gas cards each month. These were invaluable. Step two was to find out what each facility's policies were for discounts. The hospital that did my follow up mammogram, ultrasound, and biopsy offered discounts if your total was over $500.00 after insurance. In that particular case, it didn't help as my total was just under $500.00. When I checked in for my cancer surgery at Deaconness, they offered me a $135.00 discount if I paid my co-pay within 9 days. I did so. It hurt, because the co-pay was around $500.00, but dollars are dollars! My insurance covered a lot of the expenses for the surgery including the anesthesiologist, radiation department, surgeon, pathology, etc. The initial bill I discussed with the co-pay discount was just for use of the hospital facility!

Next comes all the radiation treatments and follow up doctor appointments. The radiation treatments were about $600.00 to $800.00 each, more if you saw a doctor, had a CT scan, or had X-rays taken. I filled out financial information at Cancercare and ended up getting a 100% write off on everything the insurance didn't cover. Also, during radiation, I had to stay in Spokane 4 nights a week. The American Cancer Society paid for all my stays. And they weren't in low rate motels. They put me up in the best hotels available. Sometimes I had to pay for my parking. At one hotel, they even gave me free vouchers for a breakfast buffet each day! I can't say enough about how this helped me to get rest, good nutrition, have fun, and just feel pampered sometimes.

Don't be afraid to ask, don't let pride get in the way. That's what these agencies do! I figured when all was said and done, my bills, not counting the three years of follow up appointments I've had, totaled close to $100,000. I believe I paid $2500.00 to $3000.00 out of pocket for my "castasrophic cap". I will never complain about that! The other expense is for my daily dose of Arimidex (to remove the estrogen from my body). It costs $600.00 for a 90 day supply and I have to take it for 5 years minimum. I thank God every day that my drugs are 100% covered by insurance with no co-pays. I think that would stress me out more than anything. Cancer is extremely expensive! I don't know what the chemo costs or how much a mastectomy is. I've had to have bone scans, CT Scans, and the Oncotype test I had was $6000.00. All I can say is do your homework and try every avenue to reduce the out of pocket costs. If you have to, start a Gofundme.com account or other fundraiser to try to get some donations. Do what you have to do to relieve the burden! Like I said, don't be too proud to ask.

Chapter 12
Spiritual Effects of Cancer

I include this chapter because I rely heavily on God for my strength and hope. I'd be remiss if I left Him out! I can't tell you how much it meant to me to have my church family rallying around me, always cheering me on. They sent a weeks worth of encouraging notes every week for me to open daily. They took me to lunch and got me out of the hotels for awhile. They prayed for me and over me. They understood when I just didn't have it in me to do my usual duties, like leading worship. I missed Bible studies, photography and art classes, but I did manage to get to cooking classes on the Friday afternoon when I returned home. I was determined not to let fatigue get the upper hand. Your idea of "spiritual" may be very different from mine. It is a facet of your journey and may be a very private thing. If it gives you strength, then go for it. I know that God supplies all my needs (not wants) and he kept me out of the pity-parties and into the healing parties! And God will always listen to me whether I'm ranting and raving or praising him for saving my life. Having hope and peace helps keep a great attitude. I pray you will find that hope and peace from God when or if you have to travel your own journey. If you need a place to start, read the Psalms. They are so perfect for all your hills and valleys in life.

Conclusion

It has been just over three years since my surgery to remove cancer from my right breast. It has been an eventful journey. I found out where my strengths are and how I hold up to the stresses of life. I found out how wonderful and supportive my friends and family are. I found out that my new normal is not really what I signed on for, but it is what it is and I've tried to make the best of it. I have been on mission trips to Africa three times now. I know now that life can be short, why wait to have adventures? I like to get out and travel just because. I stepped up my Ebay business. I am still taking my nasty medicine and have adjusted to the hot flashes, night sweats, insomnia and aches and pains. I would rather feel the pain of life and overcome it than be miserable. I am closer and more reliant on God and not afraid to speak up about what he has done for me. A lot of people have said that they would go through the cancer journey again because it changed the way they approach life. I do appreciate what I have much more than I did before Cancer. Don't let cancer define your life. Let it change you for the better! For me it was a big speed bump in the road. I slowed down, drove over it and continued on.

If you have any questions or comments about what you've read in this book, or a story about your journey, I'd love to hear from you!

Please write me at:

Bonnie Wilson

PO Box 722

Ione, WA 99139